Mediterranean Tasty Recipes

A Set of 50 Easy & Quick Avocado, Chicken & Soup Mediterranean Recipes

Alex Brawn

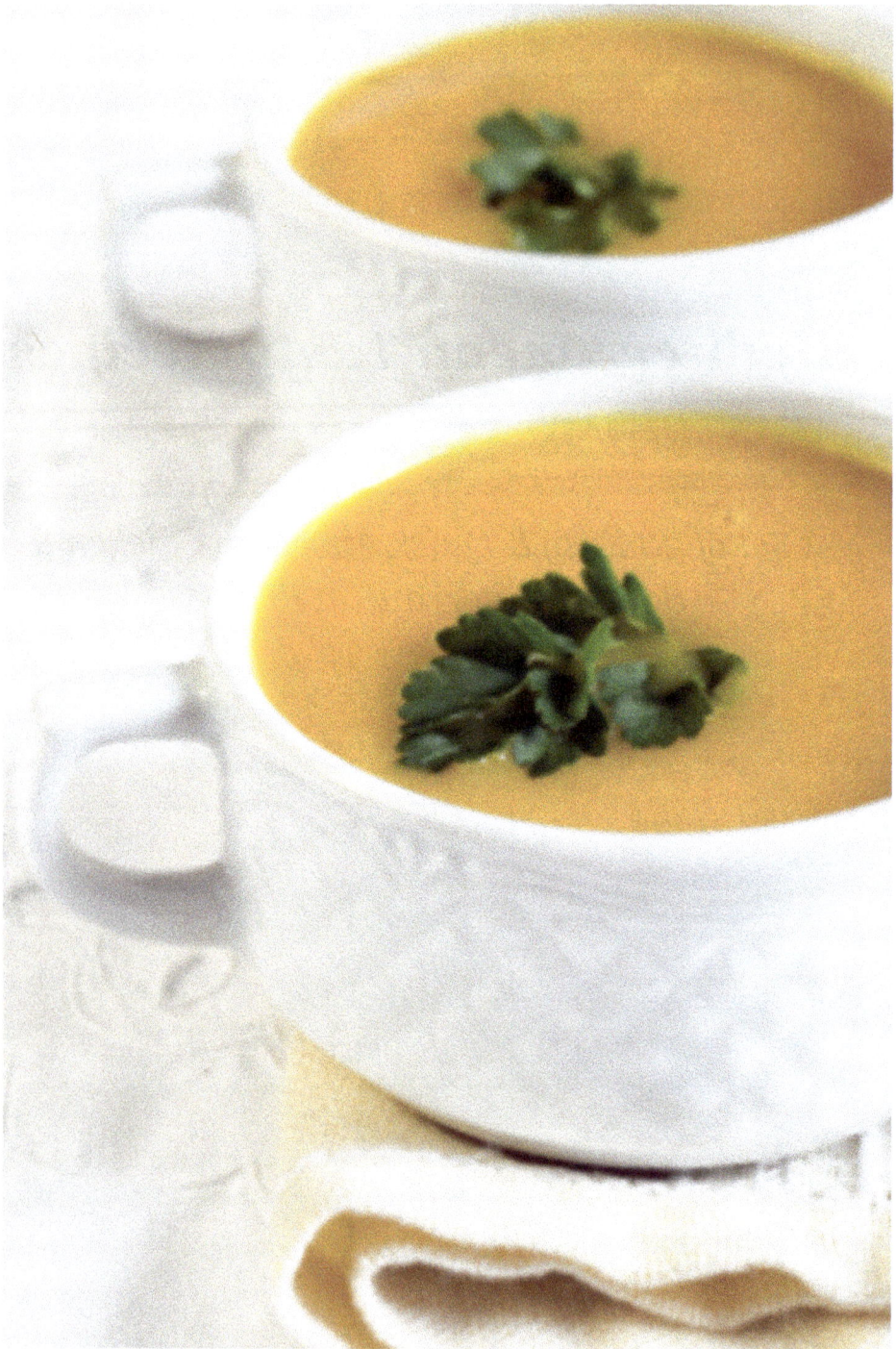

By reading this document, the reader agrees that under no circumstances is the author responsible for any losses, direct or indirect, which are incurred as a result of the use of information contained within this document, including, but not limited to, — errors, omissions, or inaccuracies.

Table of Contents

Lemon sole with chipotle and ancho chili recado 7

Salsa Verde fresco 10

Chilled avocado soup with tortilla chips 12

Charred avocado and eggs 14

Avocado and slow roasted tomatoes on the toast 16

Avocado ice cream 18

Quick flatbreads with avocado and feta 20

Smashed avocado, basil, and chicken 22

Avocado, fig, and spinach 23

Cracking cob salad 24

Avocado and peas with mashed potato 27

Avocado, pancetta, and pine nut salad 28

Roast carrot and avocado salad with orange and lemon dressing 30

Smoked salmon and avocado salad 33

Grilled chicken with charred pineapple salad 35

Salina chicken 38

Chicken tikka skewers 40

Sticky hoisin chicken 42

Sweet chicken surprise 44

Sesame butterflied chicken 46

Chicken and spring green bun cha 48

Firecracker chicken noodle salad 51

Seared turmeric chicken 53

Chicken and garlic bread kebabs 55

Piri piri chicken 57

Blackened chicken 60

Pukka yellow curry 63

Roasted chicken breast with lemony Bombay potatoes 66

CHICKEN AND SQUASH CACCIATORE 68

BARBECUED CHICKEN 70

ALL IN ONE RICE AND CHICKEN 72

MEDITERRANEAN SEA DIET SOUP RECIPES 74

TORTELLINI IN BRODO 75

SUMMERY PEA SOUP WITH TURMERIC SCALLOPS 78

HAM RIBOLLITA.. 80

MINESTRONE SOUP 82

SPICED PARSNIPS SOUP... 84

KOREAN CHICKEN HOTPOT 86

PLAYSCHOOL TOMATO SOUP... 88

THAI INSPIRED VEGETABLE BROTH 91

HOT AND SOUR CHICKEN BROTH 93

MISO SOUP WITH TOFU AND CABBAGE 95

ASIAN INSPIRED CHICKEN RICE BALLS AND BROTH 97

WATERCRESS SOUP 100

SIMPLE NOODLE SOUP... 101

FISH SOUP 103

PARSNIP, SAGE, AND WHITE BEAN SOUP....................................... 105

PUMPKIN AND GINGER SOUP 107

FRESH TOMATO BROTH... 109

SUPER TASTY MISO BROTH 111

Lemon sole with chipotle and ancho chili recado

Ingredients

- 1 ripe avocado
- Extra virgin olive oil
- 2 limes
- 4 cloves of garlic
- 2 dried chipotle chilies
- 3 spring onions
- 2 dried ancho chilies
- 1½ tablespoon of dried oregano
- 4 lemon sole
- ½ a lime
- 14 ripe cherry tomatoes
- 1 Lebanese cucumber

Directions

- Preheat the oven ready to 380°F.
- Place the unpeeled garlic in a small roasting tin and roast for 20 minutes.
- Transfer to a plate, let cool, then remove the skins.

- Place the chipotle together with the ancho chilies in a small bowl.
- Pour over boiling water to just cover, let soak for 15 minutes.
- Drain in a colander, reserving some liquid.
- Place the chilies together with the garlic, oregano, and a large pinch of sea salt in a food processor and blend to a paste.
- Add the lime juice and 4 tablespoons of the reserved liquid, blend further to combine.
- Transfer to a non-reactive bowl.
- Place the fish in the marinade, cover with Clingfilm.
- Refrigerate for 30 minutes.
- Combine chopped cucumber, spring onions, tomatoes, an avocado in a bowl with 3 tablespoons of oil and the lime juice.
- Season.
- Preheat a barbecue to a medium heat.
- Remove the fish from the refrigerator and cook, turning once, for about 3 minutes each side, brushing with marinade during cooking.

- Serve and enjoy with the avocado salad and freshly squeezed lime wedges.

Salsa Verde fresco

Ingredients

- ½ a bunch of fresh coriander
- 2 large fresh green chilies
- 2 limes
- 12 green tomatillos
- 2 onions
- 1 ripe avocado
- 1 clove of garlic

Directions

- Heat a griddle pan until screaming hot.
- Then, chargrill the chilies until their skins are black and blistered all over.
- Place the charred chilies in a bowl, cover with Clingfilm, let sit for a few minutes.
- In batches, chargrill the tomatillos with onion wedges until blackened and caramelised on all sides.
- Remove the chilies from the bowl and peel off the blackened skin.

- Place the chilies together with the onions, garlic, tomatillos, coriander leaves, and avocado on a big board.
- Chop all vegetables, mix in the lime juice and a good pinch of sea salt and black pepper.
- Blend all the ingredients in a blender until smooth.
- Drip onto eggs or on crispy chicken.
- Serve and enjoy.

Chilled avocado soup with tortilla chips

Ingredients

- 1 handful of micro garlic chives
- ½ tablespoon of olive oil
- 1 cucumber
- 4 spring onions
- 200ml of plain yoghurt
- ½ teaspoon of hot smoked paprika
- A few sprigs of fresh coriander
- 2 soft corn tortillas
- 1 large ripe avocado
- 250ml of organic vegetable stock
- 1 mild fresh green chili
- 1 lime
- Tabasco sauce
- 1 fresh red chili

Directions

- Preheat the oven to 400°F.
- Combine the oil together with the paprika, brush over both sides of the tortillas.

- Bake on a baking tray for 5 minutes, or until golden.
- Season well and set aside to cool, break into pieces.
- Blend the avocado together with the cucumber, stock, yoghurt, spring onions, coriander, and green chili until smooth.
- Then, season with lime juice, Tabasco, and a good pinch of sea salt and black pepper.
- Cover and place in the fridge to chill.
- Once the soup is chilled, serve in small bowls topped with the tortilla chips, chopped cucumber, red chili and garlic chives.
- Serve and enjoy with a drizzle of avocado oil.

Charred avocado and eggs

Ingredients

- ½ of a fresh red chili
- 4 spring onions
- A few sprigs of fresh soft herbs
- 2 tablespoons of cottage cheese
- ½ a ripe avocado
- Olive oil
- 1 sweet potato
- 1 red pepper
- 2 large free-range eggs

Directions

- Heat 1 tablespoon of olive oil over a medium-high heat.
- Add the spring onions together with the avocado and pepper, let fry for 4 minutes, or until lightly charred.
- Add peeled potatoes to the pan, toss with the charred vegetables, let fry for 3 minutes.
- Spread the vegetables evenly in the pan.
- Dig out 2 pockets.

- Crack an egg into each one, then tilt the pan so the whites run into the vegetables binding everything together.
- Season with sea salt and black pepper.
- Cover, with tin foil, lower the heat to medium−low, let the eggs cook for 5 minutes.
- Spoon the mixture onto a plate, dollop with cottage cheese and sprinkle over the herbs.

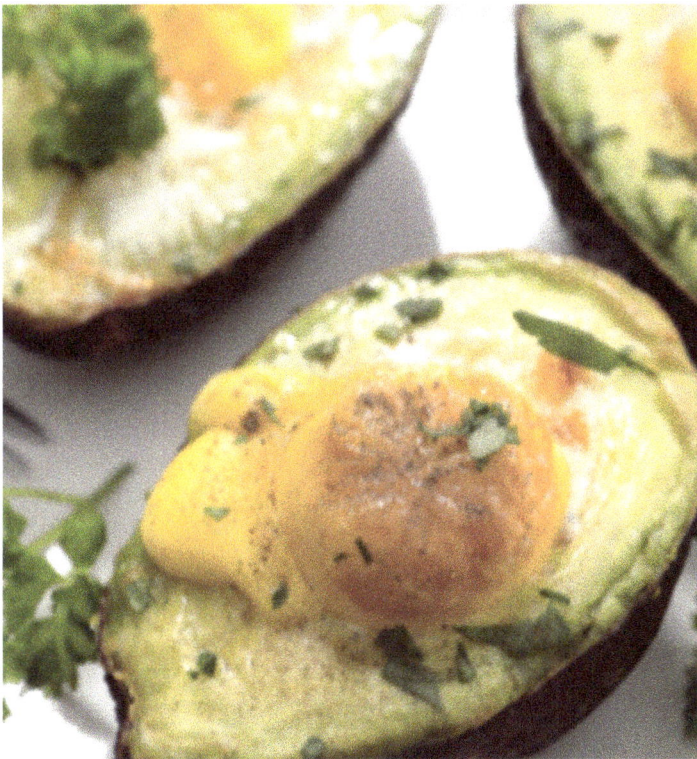

Avocado and slow roasted tomatoes on the toast

Ingredients

- 4 handfuls of rocket
- 4 plum tomatoes
- 4 slices of sourdough bread
- Olive oil
- 150g of feta cheese
- 1 bunch of fresh basil
- 1 lemon
- 3 ripe avocados

Directions

- Preheat the oven to 280°F.
- Place the tomatoes cut-side up on a baking tray.
- Season generously and drizzle with oil.
- Then, roast gently for 2 hours or until dried out.
- Pound basil leaves in a pestle and mortar with a pinch of sea salt until to foam paste.

- Pour in a good splash of oil and squeeze in the juice of ½ lemon.
- Place avocado flesh in a bowl, squeeze in the other lemon half.
- Season with salt and pepper.
- Mash with a fork to bring it all together.
- Toast the bread, then divide between 4 plates and generously spread on the avocado and top with the tomatoes.
- Serve and enjoy with crumbled feta.

Avocado ice cream

Ingredients

- 500ml of whole milk
- 200g of sugar
- 4 ripe avocados
- 2 vanilla pods
- 1 lime
- 1 lemon

Directions

- Add vanilla to saucepan with the pods.
- Add the sugar with the zest and juice.
- Bring to the boil, let simmer for a couple of minutes to dissolve the sugar.
- Remove from heat, pour into a bowl, let cool.
- Once the syrup is cool, remove the vanilla pods.
- Blend the avocado flesh with the milk to a smooth, light consistency.
- Pour it into a large baking dish, place in a freezer.

- Whisk every half hour or so until frozen and smooth.
- Serve and enjoy.

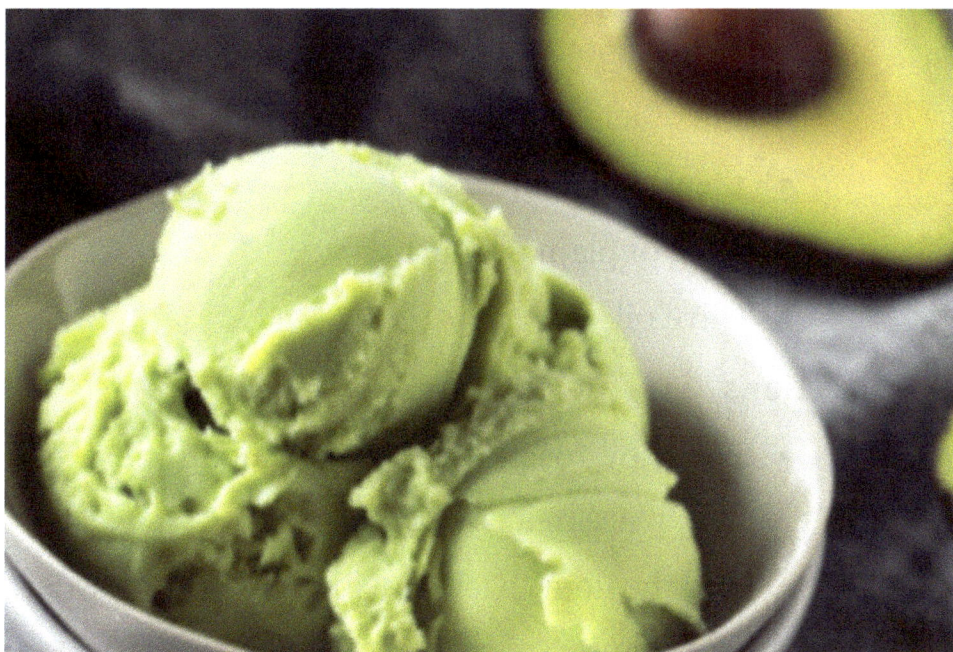

Quick flatbreads with avocado and feta

Ingredients

- 2 ripe avocados
- 250g of whole meal self-rising flour
- 1 teaspoon of rose harissa
- ¾ teaspoon of baking powder
- 75g of feta cheese
- 1 teaspoon cumin seeds
- 350g of plain yoghurt
- Olive oil

Directions

- Begin by toasting the cumin lightly in a dry pan, place in a bowl.
- Add the flour together with the baking powder, and yogurt.
- Season, and mix until dough forms.
- Turn out onto a lightly floured surface and knead until the dough together.
- Place in a lightly greased bowl, cover with a damp tea towel, let raise.

- Chop the avocado into chunks, then place in a bowl.
- Crumble in the feta with a drizzle of oil, season to taste.
- In another bowl, stir the harissa into the rest of the yoghurt.
- Divide the dough into eight balls.
- Roll each one on a lightly floured surface into an oval shape.
- Place a griddle pan over a high heat.
- Griddle each flatbread for 3 minutes, until puffed up.
- Brush the flatbread with a little oil.
- Serve and enjoy with the avocado salad and harissa yoghurt.

Smashed avocado, basil, and chicken

Ingredients

- 50g of leftover cooked chicken
- ½ of a ripe avocado
- Extra virgin olive oil
- 2 sprigs of fresh basil

Directions

- Place the avocado in a bowl and mash.
- Pick and tear in the basil leaves.
- Shred the chicken into small pieces.
- Add to the bowl.
- Then, Mix together, and add a little oil to loosen.
- Serve and enjoy.

Avocado, fig, and spinach

Ingredients

- 1 fresh fig
- ½ of a ripe avocado
- 1 large handful of baby spinach

Directions

- Place the avocado flesh in a blender.
- Add the spinach together with the fig.
- Blend to a purée.
- Taste, and adjust the thickness.
- Serve and enjoy.

Cracking cob salad

Ingredients

- 1 large pinch of sweet smoked paprika
- 2 tablespoons of Greek yoghurt
- Olive oil
- 4 slices of pancetta
- 2 large free-range eggs
- 2 free-range chicken thighs
- Extra virgin olive oil
- 1 Romaine, cos lettuce
- ½ teaspoon of Worcestershire sauce
- 1 ripe avocado
- 50ml of buttermilk
- 1 lemon
- 2 ripe tomatoes
- 1 punnet of salad cress
- 50g of Stilton
- ½ a bunch of fresh chives

Directions

- Preheat the oven to 350°F.

- Place the chicken thighs into a small roasting tray.
- Sprinkle over the paprika, and a pinch of sea salt and black pepper.
- Drizzle over a little olive oil and toss to coat.
- Let roast for 40 minutes, or until golden, laying over the pancetta for the final 10 minutes. Let cool slightly.
- Lower the eggs into a pan of vigorously simmering water and boil for 6 minutes, refreshing under cold water, peel.
- Crumble the Stilton into a large jug.
- Add chopped chives, with a drizzle of extra virgin olive oil.
- Squeeze in the lemon juice with the remaining dressing ingredients, whisk.
- Season to taste with salt and pepper, refrigerate until needed.
- Remove and discard any tatty outer leaves from the lettuce, chop the rest.
- Chop avocado, tomatoes, peeled eggs on a board and mix it together.

- Shred the chicken meat, without bones and skin.
- Add to the salad.
- Crumble over the crispy pancetta and continue chopping and mixing together.
- Transfer the salad to a platter, drizzle over the blue cheese dressing.
- Serve and enjoy.

Avocado and peas with mashed potato

Ingredients

- 1 sprig of fresh mint
- 1 potato
- 1 large ripe avocado
- 1 tablespoon of milk
- 100g of frozen peas

Directions

- Peel and dice the potato.
- Cook in boiling water for 10 minutes.
- Drain any excess water and mash with the milk.
- Cook the peas in boiling water for 3 minutes.
- Drain excess water, place into a bowl, let cool.
- Add chopped avocado to the bowl.
- Add the mint leaves and mash together.
- Serve and enjoy.

Avocado, pancetta, and pine nut salad

Ingredients

- 6 ripe avocados
- Sea salt
- 12 slices pancetta
- 50g of pine nuts
- Balsamic vinegar
- Freshly ground black pepper
- 4 big handfuls of baby spinach
- Extra virgin olive oil

Directions

- Heat a frying pan and fry the pancetta slices till crispy.
- Remove from the pan and set aside.
- In the same pan, lightly toast the pine nuts.
- Combining balsamic vinegar with olive oil.
- Season with salt and pepper.
- Lay out the avocado on a serving plate.
- Sprinkle over the spinach leaves, pancetta, and toasted pine nuts.

- Season with salt and pepper and drizzle over your dressing.
- Serve and enjoy with warm crusty bread.

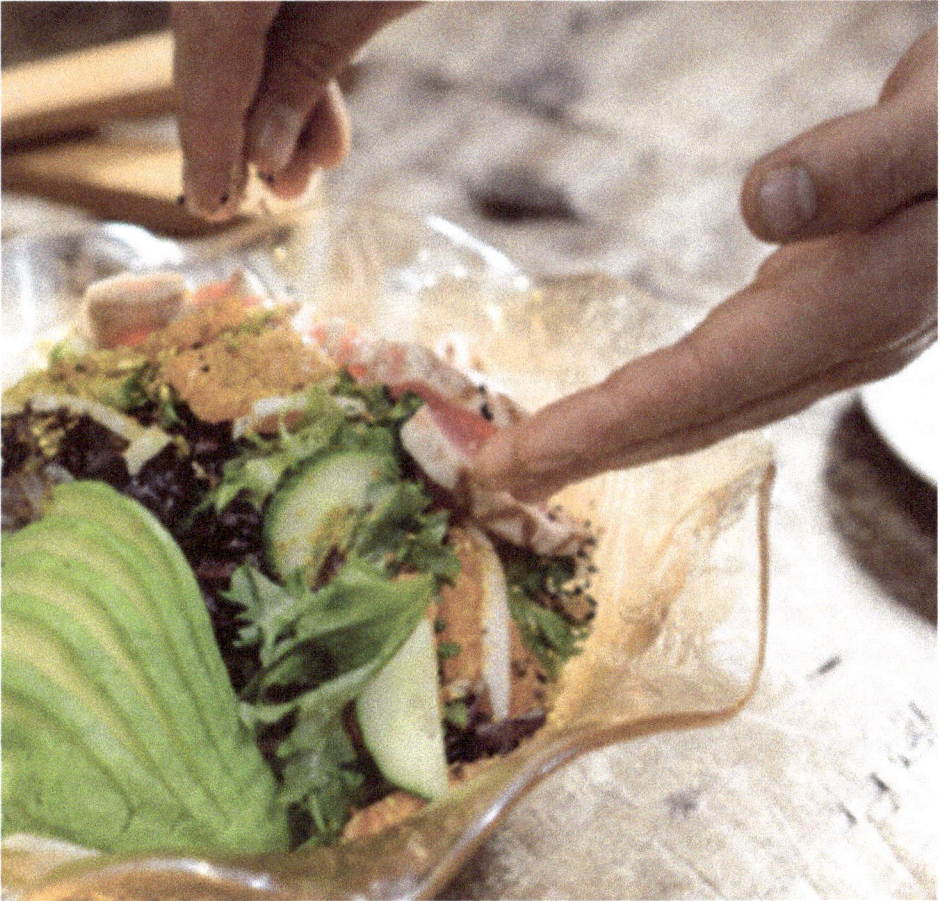

Roast carrot and avocado salad with orange and lemon dressing

Ingredients

- 2 handfuls of mixed winter salad leaves
- 500g of medium differently colored carrots
- 2 punnet cress
- 1 lemon
- 2 level teaspoons of whole cumin seeds
- 150ml of fat-free natural yoghurt
- 2 small dried chilies
- 3 ripe avocados
- 4 tablespoons of mixed seeds
- 2 cloves garlic
- Red wine vinegar
- 4 sprigs fresh thyme
- 4 x 1cm of thick slices ciabatta
- Extra virgin olive oil
- red or white wine vinegar
- 1 orange

Directions

- Preheat the oven to 350°F.

- Boil the carrots in boiling, salted water for 10 minutes.
- Drain, place into a roasting tray.
- Mash up the cumin seeds, chilies, salt and pepper in a mortar.
- Add the garlic with thyme leaves, smash up again until paste foams.
- Add enough extra virgin olive oil with vinegar to cover the past.
- Stir together, then pour over the carrots in the tray, to coat.
- Add the orange and lemon halves, cut-side down.
- Place in the preheated oven for 30 minutes.
- Remove the carrots, then add to the avocados.
- Squeeze the roasted orange and lemon juice into a bowl and add the same amount of extra virgin olive oil, with a swig of red wine vinegar.
- Season, and pour this dressing over the carrots and avocados.
- Mix together, taste and adjust the seasoning.

- Tear the toasted bread into little pieces and add to the dressed carrot and avocado.
- Serve and enjoy.

Smoked salmon and avocado salad

Ingredients

- Freshly ground black pepper
- 2 small avocados
- 1 lemon
- 200g of smoked salmon
- Sea salt
- ½ cucumber
- 2 handfuls of mixed fresh herbs
- 1 punnet cress
- 2 tablespoons of mixed seeds
- 1 loaf ciabatta
- 1 blood orange
- Extra virgin olive oil

Directions

- Heat a griddle pan until screaming hot.
- Place the sliced avocado in a bowl, squeeze over some lemon juice.
- Slice the cucumber into long, thin strips on top of the avocado.
- Then, add the herbs and cress.

- Lightly toast the seeds in a dry pan on a medium to low heat.
- Squeeze a tablespoon of juice out of the blood orange into a bowl.
- Add 3 tablespoons of extra virgin olive oil.
- Season. Mix.
- Place the ciabatta squares in the griddle pan, charring both sides.
- Once toasted, drizzle with a little of the dressing and put to one side.
- Place a square of ciabatta on each of four plates, then top each with a quarter of the smoked salmon.
- Drizzle the dressing over the salad and mix with your fingertips.
- Top the smoked salmon with the salad.
- Serve and enjoy.

Grilled chicken with charred pineapple salad

Ingredients

- ¼ of a pineapple
- ½ of an avocado
- 1 teaspoon of dried oregano
- ½ a bunch of fresh coriander
- Olive oil
- 1 fresh red chili
- 2 x 150g of free-range chicken breasts
- 2 tablespoons of pickled jalapeños
- 150 g quinoa
- 50g of white cabbage
- 2 limes
- 1 large handful of salad leaves
- 50g of natural yoghurt

Directions

- Begin by combining the oregano with olive oil in a bowl.
- Season with sea salt and black pepper.

- Place the chicken breast with olive oil in the bowl, turning until coated, then leave to one side.
- Then, cook the quinoa as per the packet Directions, drain, set aside.
- Place avocado flesh, coriander, jalapeno, and a splash of the pickling liquid and the juice of 1½ limes in a blender.
- Blend until smooth, stir through the quinoa.
- Place a griddle pan over a high heat.
- Place chopped apple on the hot griddle pan for a few minutes on each side.
- Transfer to a chopping board.
- In the same pan, griddle the chicken for 5 minutes on each side.
- Place on the chopping board, let rest and cool.
- Chop the griddled pineapple into bite-sized chunks, and the chili, then slice the chicken into thin strips.
- Divide the yoghurt among 4 plates topping with the chicken, and pineapple on one side and the dressed quinoa on the other.

- Toss the leaves and cabbage with the juice of the remaining lime, chopped chili and a little salt and pepper.
- Serve and enjoy.

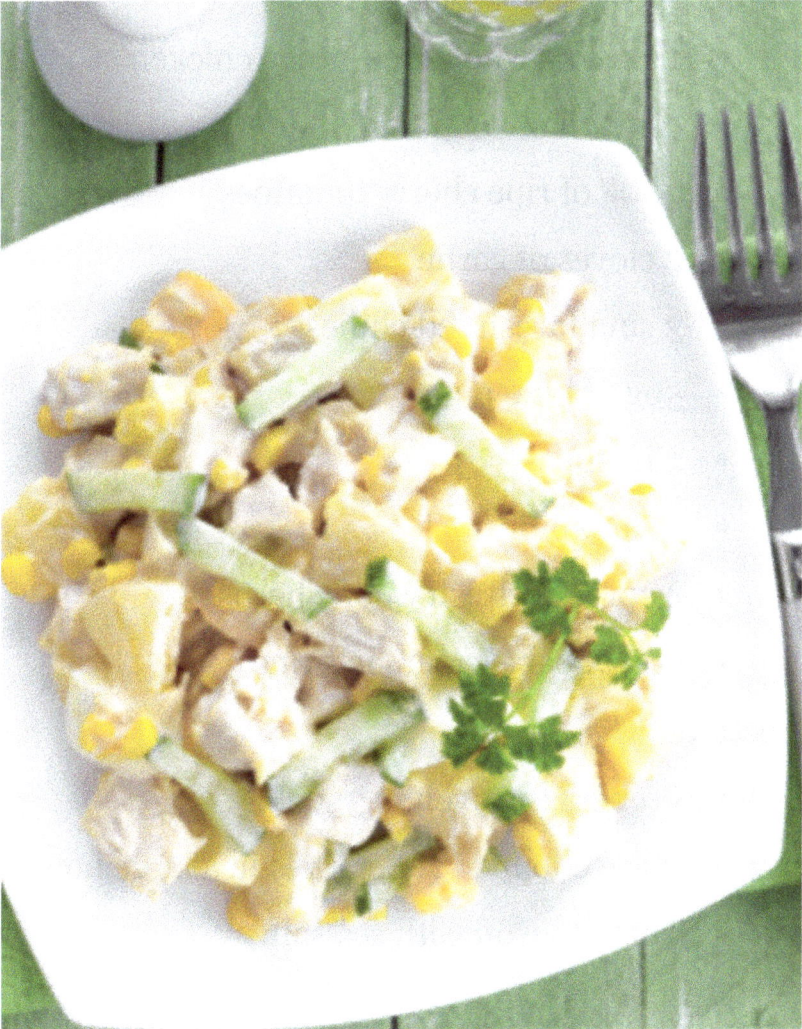

Salina chicken

Ingredients

- 4 sprigs of fresh basil
- 2 red onions
- 3 aubergines
- 1 x 1.4 kg whole free-range chicken
- olive oil
- 200g of ripe cherry tomatoes
- 2 cloves of garlic
- 3 small fresh red chilies
- 50g of pine nuts
- 2 lemons
- 1 cinnamon stick
- 4 sprigs of fresh woody herbs
- 50g of baby capers in brine

Directions

- Preheat the oven to 350°F.
- Place chopped aubergines in a large bowl.
- Then, season with sea salt.

- Drizzle the chicken pieces with olive oil, place in a large shallow pan on a medium-high heat, with skin side down turning to get golden.
- Wipe off the salt on aubergines and add to the pan, turning until lightly golden.
- Remove.
- Combine garlic with chilies, cinnamon, capers, and woody herbs add to the pan.
- Stir and fry for briefly, stir in onion, let cook for 15 minutes, stirring occasionally.
- Squeeze the tomatoes in a bowl of water, remove the seeds.
- Put the chicken and aubergines back in, drizzle over any resting juices, with half liter of water.
- Sprinkle over the pine nuts, then squeeze over the lemon juice.
- Cook at the bottom of the oven until golden.
- Pick over the basil leaves.
- Serve and enjoy with lemony couscous.

Chicken tikka skewers

Ingredients

- 3 fresh red chilies
- 2 lemons
- ½ a bunch of fresh coriander
- 2 teaspoons of tikka masala spice paste
- 2 tablespoons of natural yoghurt
- 2 little gem lettuces
- Olive oil
- ½ of a small ripe pineapple
- 2 skinless free-range chicken breasts

Directions

- Combine lemon juice, olive oil, paste, and yogurt, then mix well.
- Add sliced pineapple, chilies, sliced chicken to the bowl with the marinade.
- Toss together to coat, place in the fridge to marinate overnight.
- Remove the chicken and pineapple mixture from the fridge.
- Remove and tear the chili into smaller pieces.

- Starting with the chicken, thread the ingredients onto skewers, alternating between the ingredients.
- Pour any remaining marinade over the top and drizzle with a little oil.
- Put a dry pan on a medium heat, then add the skewers, let cook for 10 minutes, turning occasionally, season with a little sea salt.
- Roughly shave the chicken, pineapple and chili from the skewers with a knife, scatter over the reserved lemon zest and pick over the coriander leaves.
- Slice the remaining lemon into wedges for squeezing over.
- Serve and enjoy with the lettuce and yoghurt.

Sticky hoisin chicken

Ingredients

- 3 regular oranges
- 2 x 200g of free-range chicken legs
- 2 heaped tablespoons of hoisin sauce
- 2 fresh mixed-color chilies
- 8 spring onions

Directions

- Preheat the oven ready to 350°F.
- Place an ovenproof frying pan on a high heat.
- Pull off the chicken skin, put both skin and legs into the pan.
- Season with sea salt and black pepper, letting the fat render out and the chicken get golden, turning halfway.
- Toss the white spring onions into the pan, after which transfer to the oven for 15 minutes.
- Place chilies and green spring onions into a bowl of ice-cold water to curl.
- Arrange sliced oranges on a plates.

- Remove the chicken skin and soft spring onions from the pan. Set aside.
- Cook the chicken until tender and cooked through.
- In a bowl, loosen the hoisin with a splash of red wine vinegar, spoon over the chicken.
- Sit the chicken and soft spring onions on top and crack over the crispy skin.
- Serve and enjoy.

Sweet chicken surprise

Ingredients

- 4 sprigs of fresh tarragon
- 2 x 200g of free-range chicken legs
- 100ml of red vermouth
- 1 bulb of garlic
- 250g of mixed-color seedless grapes

Directions

- Start by preheating the oven to 350°F.
- Then, place an ovenproof frying pan over high heat.
- Rub the chicken with ½ a tablespoon of olive oil.
- Then, season with sea salt and black pepper and place skin side down in the pan.
- Fry for a couple of minutes until golden.
- Squash the unpeeled garlic cloves, add with grapes to the pan.
- Turn the chicken skin side up, then pour in the vermouth.

- Transfer to the oven, let roast for 40 minutes, or until the chicken tender.
- Add a splash of water to the pan and to pick up all the sticky bits.
- Serve and enjoy.

Sesame butterflied chicken

Ingredients

- 2 tablespoons of natural yoghurt
- 1 tablespoon of low-salt soy sauce
- 100g of fine rice noodles
- 2cm piece of ginger
- 2 x 120g of skinless free-range chicken breasts
- 1 tablespoon of peanut butter
- 2 teaspoons of sesame seeds
- 2 limes
- Groundnut oil
- 4 spring onions
- ½ of a Chinese cabbage
- 200g of sugar snap peas
- 1 fresh red chili

Directions

- Place your griddle pan over high heat.
- Then, in a bowl, cover the noodles with boiling kettle water.
- Rub with 1 teaspoon of groundnut oil on chicken opened up.

- Season with a small pinch of sea salt and black pepper.
- Let griddle for 8 minutes, turning halfway.
- Trim the spring onions and rattle them through the finest slicer on your food processor with the Chinese cabbage, sugar snap peas and chili.
- Dress with the juice of 1 lime and the soy sauce.
- In a separate small bowl, mix the peanut butter together with the yoghurt and the juice of the remaining lime, ginger, mix.
- Slice the chicken on a board, toast lightly with the sesame seeds in the residual heat of the griddle pan.
- Sprinkle over the chicken.
- Drain the noodles, divide between plates with the chicken, slaw and peanut sauce, mix.
- Serve and enjoy.

Chicken and spring green bun cha

Ingredients

- ½ a bunch of fresh mint
- 2 spring onions
- 100g frozen edamame beans
- 1 stick of lemongrass
- 3 tablespoons of vegetable oil
- 5cm piece of ginger
- 1 large fresh red chili
- 200g of baby spinach
- 1½ tablespoons of sesame oil
- 1 tablespoon of low-salt soy sauce
- 150g of broad beans
- 2 tablespoons of runny honey
- 2 tablespoons of hoisin sauce
- 2 limes
- 4 free-range skinless chicken thighs
- 1 tablespoon of rice wine vinegar
- 1 x 225g packet of vermicelli
- 2 large shallots
- ½ a bunch of fresh Thai basil

Directions

- Preheat the oven to 400°F.
- Place the lemongrass in a large bowl together with the sesame oil, soy sauce, the zest from 1 lime, honey, hoisin sauce, and the juice from 2 limes. Mix, pour half into a small bowl.
- Add the chicken to the large bowl, stir and let marinate.
- Add the rice wine vinegar to the small bowl.
- Cook defrosted beans in a pan of boiling water for 2 minutes.
- Drain and rinse under cold water. Set aside.
- Cook the vermicelli according to the packet Directions, drain.
- Place the chicken in a small roasting tin lined with tinfoil, move it in the oven heated for 30 minutes.
- Then, heat olive oil in a small, pan over a medium-high heat.
- When hot enough, add the shallots, let cook for 5 minutes.

- Remove, set aside on a tray lined with kitchen paper.
- Combine the noodles together with the remaining dressing, spring onion, broad beans, baby spinach, and herbs.
- Top with the chicken, garnished with the shallots.
- Serve and enjoy.

Firecracker chicken noodle salad

Ingredients

- 1 tablespoon of sweet chili sauce
- 1 tablespoon of coriander oil
- 50g of rice noodles
- ½ tablespoon of low-salt soy sauce
- 1 lime
- 100g of cooked free-range chicken
- ¼ of a cucumber
- 1 carrot
- ½ tablespoon of runny honey
- 1 baby gem lettuce
- 1 small handful of sugar snaps
- A few sprigs of fresh mint
- 1 pinch of mixed seeds

Directions

- Cook the noodles as instructed on the package.
- Combine the shredded chicken with the cooked noodles and coriander oil in a bowl.
- Add all the remaining salad ingredients, toss to combine.

- Place the sweet chili sauce together with the soy and honey in a small jar. Chill in the lunchbox.
- Squeeze in the lime juice, secure the lid, keep in the lunchbox.
- Shake the jam jar to mix the ingredients then dress the salad.
- Close your lunchbox, shake to coat.
- Serve and enjoy chilled or at room temperature.

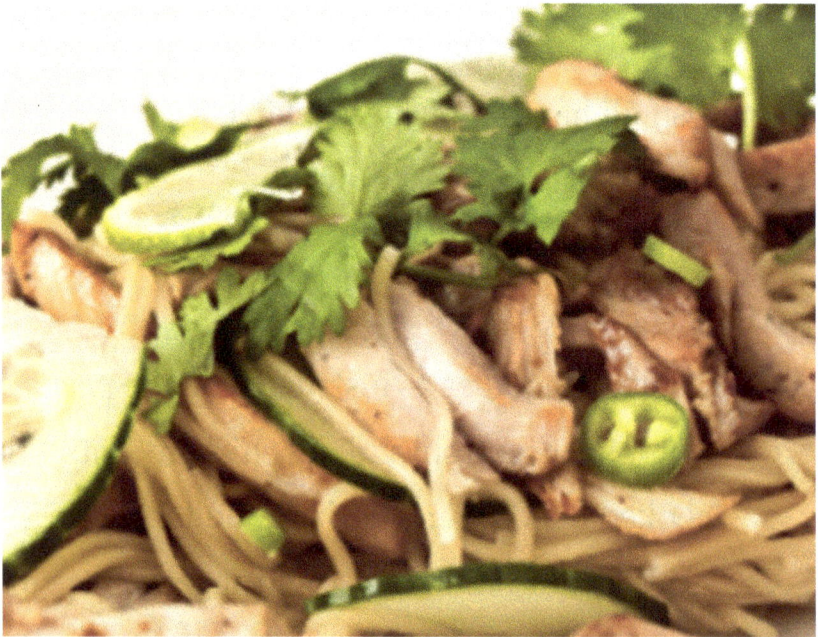

Seared turmeric chicken

Ingredients

- Olive oil
- 200g of seasonal greens
- 2 x 120g of skinless chicken breasts
- 150g of whole wheat couscous
- 2 tablespoons of natural yoghurt
- 2 sprigs of fresh oregano
- ½ a bunch of fresh mint
- 1 lemon
- 1 tablespoon of blanched hazelnuts
- 2 large roasted peeled red peppers in brine
- Hot chili sauce
- 1 level teaspoon of ground turmeric

Directions

- Combine the oregano leaves, turmeric, olive oil, pinch of salt and black pepper to make a marinade.
- Then, toss the chicken in the marinade and leave aside.

- In a boiling water, blanch the greens until tender enough to eat, drain, reserving the water.
- In a bowl, cover the couscous with boiling greens water, season with a plate on top for 10 minutes.
- Stir chopped mint leaves into the fluffy couscous with the juice of half a lemon.
- Toast the hazelnuts in a large dry frying pan on a medium-high heat.
- Remove, and crush in mortar once lightly golden.
- Return the frying pan to a high heat, let the chicken cook for 4 minutes on each side, turning halfway.
- Serve the chicken with the couscous, peppers, greens and yoghurt, scattered with the hazelnuts, with a lemon wedge on the side.
- Enjoy.

Chicken and garlic bread kebabs

Ingredients

- 1 lemon
- 2 sprigs of fresh rosemary
- 2 blood oranges
- 1 tablespoon of balsamic vinegar
- 2 cloves of garlic
- Extra virgin olive oil
- 1 tablespoon white wine vinegar
- 20g of feta cheese
- 8 fresh bay leaves
- Cayenne pepper
- 2 x 120g skinless chicken breasts
- 2 thick slices of whole meal bread
- 100g of baby spinach

Directions

- Mash up rosemary with a pinch of sea salt in a pestle and mortar. Peel and crush in the garlic, then muddle in 1 tablespoon of oil, the vinegar and a generous pinch of cayenne.

- Place chopped chicken and bread in a bowl, toss to mix well with the marinade until evenly coated.
- Place the frying pan on a medium-high heat.
- Then, lay the skewers in the pan, let cook for 5 minutes on each side.
- Dress the spinach with a squeeze of lemon juice and a drizzle of olive oil.
- Organize on the plates with the blood oranges and drizzle with the balsamic.
- Serve and enjoy topped with the kebabs and lemon wedges.

Piri piri chicken

Ingredients

- 1.3kg of chicken
- 3 sprigs of fresh thyme
- 4 cloves of garlic
- Olive oil
- 2 red onions
- 4 ripe mixed-color tomatoes
- 6 fresh mixed-color chilies
- Red wine vinegar
- Extra virgin olive oil
- 750g of sweet potatoes
- 2 teaspoons of smoked paprika
- 2 tablespoons of fine semolina
- 1 x 200g jar of pickled jalapeños
- 1 bunch of fresh coriander

Directions

- Combine thyme leaves, garlic, paprika, and a pinch of sea salt in a pestle and mortar.
- Blend to foam paste, add 2 tablespoons of olive oil.

- Rub the marinade on the chicken.
- Cover properly, and refrigerate to marinate overnight or more than, two hours, if one has no time.
- Preheat the oven to 350°F.
- Then, place a large griddle pan over a high heat.
- Place unpeeled onions and tomatoes, chilies, and unpeeled garlic on the hot griddle.
- Let, grill for 10 minutes, turning regularly.
- Remove the garlic skins and peel the onions.
- Add every vegetable to a food processor with a splash of red wine vinegar and extra virgin olive oil.
- Blend until smooth, adjusting with water if too thick.
- Season, and adjust.
- Return the griddle pan to a high heat, then add the marinated chicken and sear all over for 10 minutes, turning regularly.
- Then, transfer to a roasting tray, put in the hot oven for 45 minutes.

- Toss the sweet potatoes with the paprika, semolina, extra virgin olive oil, a small pinch of salt and black pepper.
- Spread the wedges out on 2 large baking trays.
- Place in the oven for 30 minutes, or until tender and crisp.
- Drain and add the jalapeños to a food processor with a splash of the pickling juice.
- Tear in the coriander with a splash of extra virgin olive oil.
- Blend until smooth.
- Serve the roast chicken with piri piri sauce, sweet potato wedges and a little jalapeño salsa.
- Enjoy.

Blackened chicken

Ingredients

- Olive oil
- 1 heaped teaspoon of ground allspice
- 300g of quinoa
- 2 x 200g of skinless chicken breasts
- 2 mixed-color peppers
- 1 fresh red chili
- 4 tablespoons of fat-free yoghurt
- 1 punnet cress
- 100g of baby spinach
- 4 spring onions
- 1 bunch of fresh coriander
- 1 bunch of fresh mint
- 1 large ripe mango
- 2 limes
- 2 tablespoons of extra virgin olive oil
- 1 ripe avocado
- 50g of feta cheese
- 1 heaped teaspoon of smoked paprika

Directions

- Firstly, put the quinoa into the pan and generously cover with boiling water.
- Combine the chili together with the spinach, spring onions, leafy mint, and coriander into the processor, blend until finely chopped.
- Toss the chicken with sea salt, black pepper, the allspice, and paprika on a greaseproof pan.
- Fold over the paper, then flatten the chicken.
- Place into the frying pan with 1 tablespoon of olive oil, turning after 4 minutes.
- Then, add peppers to the frying pan, tossing regularly.
- Drain the quinoa, place on to a serving board.
- Toss with the blended spinach mixture, squeeze over the lime juice.
- Add the extra virgin olive oil, mix and season to taste.
- Sprinkle the mango chunks and cooked peppers over the quinoa.
- Scoop curls of avocado flesh over the salad.

- Slice up the chicken, toss the slices in any juices, then add to the salad.
- Crumble over the feta, scatter over the remaining coriander leaves.
- Serve and enjoy with a dollop of yoghurt.

Pukka yellow curry

Ingredients

- Natural yoghurt
- 2 onions
- 1 teaspoon of tomato puree
- 1 level teaspoon of ground turmeric
- 4 cloves of garlic
- 1 lemon
- 2 teaspoons of curry powder
- 5cm piece of ginger
- 2 yellow peppers
- 1 organic chicken stock cube
- Olive oil
- 1 mug of basmati rice
- 2 fresh red chilies
- ½ a bunch of fresh coriander
- 1 teaspoon of runny honey
- 8 chicken drumsticks
- 1 x 400 g tin of chickpeas

Directions

- Place 1 onion, pepper, garlic, and ginger into a food processor.
- Then, crumble in the stock cube with the chili, coriander stalks, honey, and spices. Blend until paste forms.
- Place a large casserole pan on a medium-high heat.
- Fry the chicken drumsticks with a splash of olive oil for 10 minutes, turning occasionally.
- Remove the chicken to a plate, leaving the pan on the heat.
- Add the remaining onion and pepper to the pan, let cook briefly.
- Then place in the paste, let cook for 5 minutes.
- Pour in 500ml of boiling water.
- Drain the chickpeas, add with the tomato puree and a pinch of sea salt and black pepper, then stir.
- Return the chicken to the pan, cover, simmer gently for 45 minutes over low heat.

- Place in 1 mug of rice with 2 mugs of boiling water into a pan with a pinch of salt let simmer for 12 minutes covered.
- Serve and enjoy.

Roasted chicken breast with lemony Bombay potatoes

Ingredients

- Olive oil
- 200g of potatoes
- A few sprigs of fresh coriander
- 2cm piece of ginger
- ¼ teaspoon of ground turmeric
- ½ red pepper
- 1 free-range chicken breast
- ½ teaspoon of ground cumin
- 1 lemon

Directions

- Preheat the oven to 400°F.
- Cook the potatoes in boiling salted water for 6 minutes, drain and steam dry.
- Add the turmeric, cumin, coriander leaves, ginger, pepper, grate lemon zest to a bowl.
- Squeeze a little juice from the remainder of the lemon into the bowl.

- Shake the potatoes up in the colander, add to the bowl with the chicken.
- Drizzle with olive oil.
- Season with sea salt and black pepper, toss to coat.
- Remove the chicken from the bowl, place the potato mixture into a baking dish.
- Spread out into a single layer topping with the lemon slices, then drape over the chicken.
- Drizzle with olive oil, cook in the middle of the oven for 25 minutes.
- Serve and enjoy.

Chicken and squash cacciatore

Ingredients

- 8 black olives
- 250ml of Chianti
- 1 onion
- 4 chicken thighs, bone in
- 1 leek
- 4 cloves of garlic
- 200g of seeded whole meal bread
- Olive oil
- 2 fresh bay leaves
- 2 sprigs of fresh rosemary
- ½ a butternut squash
- 100g of shell nut mushrooms
- 2 rashers of smoked pancetta
- 2 x 400g tins of plum tomatoes

Directions

- Preheat your oven to 375°F.
- Place a large ovenproof casserole pan on a medium heat.

- Place sliced pancetta, rosemary leaves, 1 tablespoon of olive oil, onion, garlic, bay leaves, and leek in the pan. Stir regularly for 10 minutes.
- Add the stalk with the whole mushrooms, squash to the pan.
- Remove and discard the chicken skin and add the chicken to the pan.
- Pour in the wine, let reduce slightly.
- Add the tomatoes and break them up with a wooden spoon.
- Half-fill each tin with water, swirl about, pour into the pan, mix.
- Destone and poke the olives into the stew.
- Bring to a gentle simmer.
- Transfer to the oven, let cook for 1 hour.
- Season, and adjust accordingly.
- Serve and enjoy.

Barbecued chicken

Ingredients

- 24 ripe cherry tomatoes
- 2 sprigs of fresh rosemary
- Olive oil
- 1 lemon
- 1 teaspoon of wholegrain mustard
- 400g of green beans
- 4 skinless chicken breasts
- Extra virgin olive oil

Directions

- Preheat the oven to 200°F.
- Place rosemary leaves and a pinch of sea salt in a mortar, bash well.
- Add the grated lemon zest and squeeze in half the juice with 2 tablespoons of olive oil.
- Open the chicken breast and flatten
- Pour the rosemary marinade over the chicken, let marinate briefly.
- Mix the mustard with the remaining lemon juice and more extra virgin olive oil.

- Place the tomatoes onto a tray, season, roast for 20 minutes.
- Cook the beans in a pan of boiling salted water for 5 minutes.
- Drain, toss in the mustard dressing, add the roasted tomatoes.
- Preheat a barbecue.
- Barbecue the chicken breasts for 5 minutes, turning regularly.
- Serve and enjoy with beans and tomatoes.

All in one rice and chicken

Ingredients

- 250g of long-grain rice
- Olive oil
- 2 teaspoons of ground coriander
- 1 tablespoon of runny honey
- 2 chicken legs
- A few sprigs of fresh coriander
- 2 chicken thighs
- 1 onion
- 1 clove of garlic
- 1 heaped teaspoon of ground cumin
- 150g of dates

Directions

- Heat a splash of olive oil, then brown the chicken legs and thighs in a pan. Remove.
- Add diced onion, let sweet, then add crushed garlic with the spices in the same a pan.
- Let cook for 2 minutes, stir in the rice together with the dates, honey, and browned chicken.

- Cover with water, let boil, then let simmer, for 30 minutes covered over low heat.
- Season with sea salt and black pepper.
- Scatter over the chopped coriander leaves.
- Serve and enjoy.

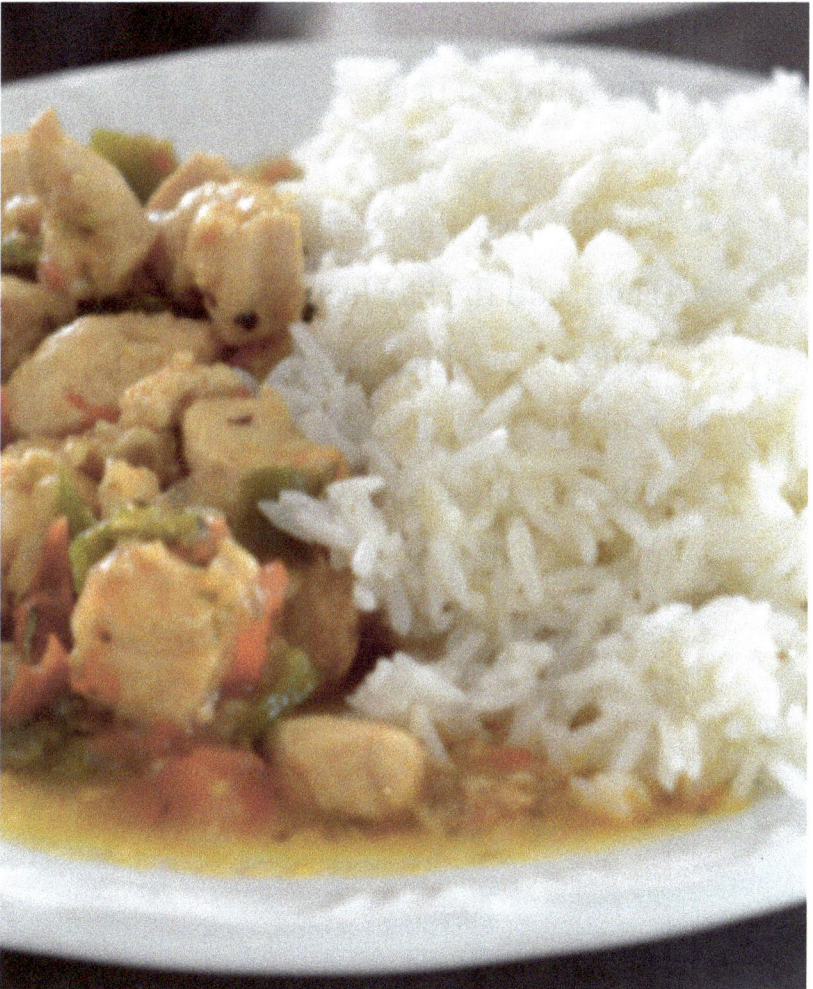

Mediterranean Sea diet soup recipes

Spinach and tortellini soup

Ingredients

- 1 large handful of spinach
- 200g of tortellini
- 1-liter organic chicken
- 2 fresh bay leaves
- 50g of frozen peas

Directions

- Firstly, pour the stock into a large pan.
- Then, add the bay leaves, bring to the boil.
- Add the tortellini, let cook for 4 minutes.
- Add the peas, let cook for a further 3 minutes.
- Add the spinach and cook until wilted.
- Place into bowls.
- Serve and enjoy with crusty bread.

Tortellini in brodo

Ingredients

- 50g of Parmesan cheese
- 150g of beef shank bones
- 75g of prosciutto di Parma
- olive oil
- 1 pinch of ground nutmeg
- 300g of free-range chicken thighs and drumsticks
- ½ of an onion
- 50g of mortadella di Bologna
- 1 stick of celery
- 1 carrot
- 200g tipo flour
- 300g of beef brisket
- 2 large free-range eggs
- 75g pf lean minced beef

Directions

- Add carrots, chicken, unpeeled onion, celery, and a pinch of salt to a stockpot, cover with enough water.

- Bring to boil, then cover, let simmer for 4 hours as you skim occasionally.
- Blend the tipo flour with eggs in a food processor until soft but firm dough, wrap in Clingfilm, let rest for 30 minutes.
- Heat a little olive oil, season the mince and fry until cooked through.
- Drain any water, let cool.
- Transfer to a blender with the prosciutto, mortadella, grated parmesan, and nutmeg. Blend until fine.
- Divide the dough into 8 pieces. Use a pasta machine to roll out 1 piece into a long, flat, thin strip. Slice into 3cm squares.
- Lightly dust a tray with flour.
- Place a ¼ of a teaspoon of filling in the middle of a square of pasta.
- Fold the pasta over into a triangle, and press to seal.
- Repeat until you have used all the rolled-out dough.

- Strain the stock and discard the meat and vegetables.
- Taste and adjust the seasoning accordingly.
- Bring to the boil, add tortellini and cook for about 3 minutes.
- Serve and enjoy.

Summery pea soup with turmeric scallops

Ingredients

- ¼ teaspoon of ground turmeric
- 2 teaspoons of tamarind paste
- 1 bunch of spring onions
- 1 clove of garlic
- 175g of queen scallops
- 5cm piece of ginger
- ½ teaspoon of mustard seeds
- 1 fresh green Bird's-eye chili
- ½ a lime
- 1 teaspoon of cumin seeds
- 10 fresh curry leaves
- Groundnut oil
- 3 fresh curry leaves
- 800ml of organic vegetable
- 450g of fresh or frozen peas
- ½ teaspoon of jiggery

Directions

- Toast the cumin seeds, add 2 tablespoons of oil with the spring onions, garlic, ginger, chili, and curry leaves.
- Fry until sizzling, then pour in the stock and bring to the boil.
- Add the peas, let simmer for 5 minutes.
- Stir in the jiggery with the tamarind paste.
- Season to taste.
- Blender to purée until smooth. Set aside.
- The heat 1 tablespoon of olive oil over a high heat.
- Add the mustard seeds and stir continuously to form soup.
- Mix in the turmeric with the curry leaves, scallops, fry briefly on each side, until beginning to brown.
- Reheat the soup, taste, and adjust.
- Serve and enjoy.

Ham ribollita

Ingredients

- 150g leftover ham
- 300g of cavolo Nero
- 1 onion
- 750ml of organic stock
- 2 cloves of garlic
- 1 x 400g tin of cannellini beans
- 2 sticks of celery
- 1 carrot
- Olive oil
- 2 teaspoons of fennel seeds
- 100g of spinach
- 1 x 400g tin of plum tomatoes

Directions

- Heat a drizzle of olive oil over a medium heat.
- Then, add celery, carrot, onion, garlic, and fennel seeds, and season.
- Cook over low heat for 10 minutes covered, until golden brown, stirring regularly.

- Mash most of the cannellini beans, add to the pan with the liquid from the tin, tomatoes, and the stock.
- Let simmer for more 10 minutes.
- Stir in chopped cavelo Nero, torn ham, and remaining beans, and spinach.
- Simmer until the greens have cooked down.
- Serve and enjoy.

Minestrone soup

Ingredients

- 2 x 400g tins of beans
- 100g of dried pasta
- 4 rashers of smoked streaky bacon
- Olive oil
- Parmesan cheese
- 1 clove of garlic
- 2 small onions
- Extra virgin olive oil
- 1 x 400g tin of quality plum tomatoes
- 2 fresh bay leaves
- 2 carrots
- 2 sticks of celery
- 2 large handfuls of seasonal greens
- 1 vegetable stock cube

Directions

- Heat a large shallow casserole pan on a medium-high heat.
- Sprinkle sliced bacon into the pan with 1 tablespoon of olive oil, stirring occasionally.

- Add the chopped garlic, onion, and bay to the pan when the bacon turns golden.
- Add chopped celery and carrots to the pan.
- Remove and finely chop any tough stalks from your greens and add to the pan.
- Let cook for 15 minutes, stirring regularly.
- Pour in the tinned tomatoes with 1 tin's worth of water.
- Add the beans together with the juice and a pinch of sea salt and black pepper.
- Sprinkle greens into the pan, top with boiling water, then add the pasta.
- Cover, let simmer for 15 minutes.
- Taste, and adjust the seasoning accordingly.
- Serve and enjoy with parmesan cheese.

Spiced parsnips soup

Ingredients

- 800g of parsnips
- 4 sprigs of fresh coriander
- 1 onion
- 4 tablespoons of natural yoghurt
- 2 cloves of garlic
- 1.5 liters of organic vegetable stock
- 5cm piece of ginger
- Olive oil
- 4 uncooked poppadoms
- 1 teaspoon of cumin seeds
- Garam masala
- 200g of red split lentils

Directions

- Start by preheating your oven ready to 350°F.
- Place the parsnips and onions in a large pan over a medium heat with 1 tablespoon of olive oil.
- Cook covered for 20 minutes, stirring occasionally.

- Add the garlic together with the ginger, scatter over the cumin seeds, 1 teaspoon of garam masala and the lentils.
- Cook for 5 more minutes.
- Roughly snap in the uncooked poppadoms, stock, let simmer for 20 minutes.
- Blanch reserved parsnips for 30 seconds in fast boiling water, drain and pat dry.
- Season with sea salt.
- Spread out in a single layer over a couple of oiled baking trays.
- Let roast for 15 minutes.
- Pick over the coriander leaves, sprinkle with a little garam masala, and top with the parsnip crisps.
- Serve and enjoy.

Korean chicken hotpot

Ingredients

- 1 lime
- 150g of shiitake mushrooms
- 2 teaspoons of sesame oil
- 2 teaspoons of Korean chili paste
- 2 large carrots
- 250g of whole wheat noodles
- 1 bunch of spring onions
- 350g of firm silken tofu
- 2 teaspoons of sesame seeds
- 200g of kimchee
- 4 free-range chicken thighs
- 1 liter of organic chicken stock
- 1 teaspoon of low-salt soy sauce

Directions

- Char the mushrooms in a casserole pan on a medium heat for 5 minutes, turning half way.
- Remove the mushrooms to a plate, add the chicken and carrots to the pan.
- Let cook for 10 minutes, stirring regularly.

- Pour in the stock, bring to the boil, let simmer for 20 minutes.
- Stir in the spring onions with mushrooms, tofu, soy sauce, and chili paste.
- Let simmer again for 20 minutes.
- Stir through the kimchee.
- Cook the noodles according to the packet Directions, drain.
- Toss with the sesame oil and seeds.
- Taste the broth, and adjust the seasoning.
- Serve and enjoy.

Playschool tomato soup

Ingredients

- 150g of pasta
- 2 x 400g tins of quality plum tomatoes
- 2 carrots
- 8 slices of sourdough
- 2 leeks
- 2 sticks of celery
- 2 onions
- Extra virgin olive oil
- 125g of mature Cheddar cheese
- 6 large ripe tomatoes
- 4 cloves of garlic
- Olive oil
- 1 organic chicken stock cube
- ½ a bunch of fresh basil

Directions

- Preheat the oven to 375°F.
- Toss all the vegetables and the tomatoes together in a deep roasting tray, season with season well with extra virgin olive oil.

- Spread the vegetables into 1 layer, place in the oven for 40 minutes.
- Bash pickled leaves to a paste, with a pinch of sea salt, until smooth.
- Toss the basil stalks into the roasted vegetable, squeeze the garlic out of its skins into the tray, add tinned tomatoes and stock.
- Bring to a boil over a medium heat.
- Lower the heat, let simmer for about 15 minutes, or until thickened.
- Remove the tray, pulse the soup until smooth.
- Return the soup to the hob over a medium heat.
- Then, season to taste and stir in the pasta.
- Simmer for 5 minutes, or until the pasta is cooked.
- Toast the bread, coarsely grate the cheese.
- Place the hot soup into bowls, scatter over most of the cheese, stir through.
- Top with a piece of toast, scatter over the remaining cheese, and finish with a drizzle of the basil oil.

- Serve and enjoy.

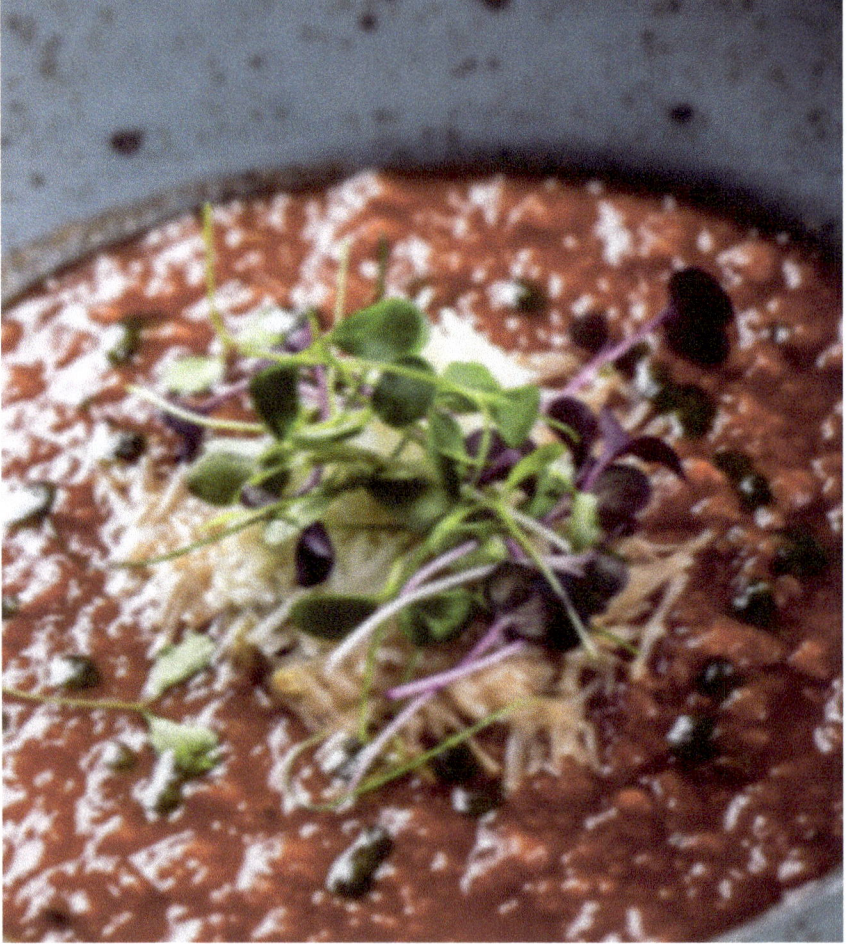

Thai inspired vegetable broth

Ingredients

- 1 teaspoon of fish sauce
- 3 cloves of garlic
- 5cm piece of ginger
- 800ml of clear organic vegetable stock
- 1 small punned shiso cress
- 200g of mixed Asian greens
- 1 lime
- 2 spring onions
- 1 fresh red chili
- 1 teaspoon of soy sauce
- 5 sprigs of fresh Thai basil
- 1 stick of lemongrass
- 2-star anise

Directions

- Bash the lemongrass on a chopping board with a rolling pin until it breaks open.
- Add to a large saucepan together with the garlic, ginger, and star anise.

- Pour in the vegetable stock in a pan over a high heat.
- Bring let boil briefly, lower heat and gently simmer for 30 minutes.
- Place in Asian veggies, let cook until they are wilted few minutes to cook time.
- Serve the broth in deep bowls.
- Seasoned with fish sauce and soy sauce, sprinkle with the herbs.
- Serve and enjoy.

Hot and sour chicken broth

Ingredients

- 2 shallots
- 1 large handful of beansprouts
- Fish sauce
- 3 sticks of lemongrass
- 5cm of ginger
- 1.75 liters light organic chicken
- 2 cloves of garlic
- 3 limes
- 2 fresh red chilies
- ½ a bunch of fresh coriander
- Groundnut oil
- 1 bunch of spring onions
- 2 free-range chicken breasts

Directions

- Gently sweat the shallots in a splash of oil until soft.
- Place in the lemongrass together with the ginger, stock, most of the chili and garlic, and fry for 1 minute.

- Add the chicken and simmer for 8 minutes, or until the chicken is cooked through.
- Then, add a splash of fish sauce and squeeze in the lime juice.
- Taste, and adjust seasoning with fish sauce, lime juice or chili.
- Add the coriander, beansprouts, and spring onions.
- Serve and enjoy.

Miso soup with tofu and cabbage

Ingredients

- ½ savoy cabbage
- 100g of silken tofu
- 750ml of organic chicken
- 1 carrot
- 3cm piece of ginger
- Low-salt soy sauce
- 2 cloves of garlic
- 2 tablespoons of miso paste
- 1 fresh red chili

Directions

- Pour the stock into a pan, bring to a boil.
- Add ginger, garlic, and chili to the stock, cover and simmer for 5 minutes.
- Add carrots and cabbage to the pan, cover and simmer for 4 more minutes, or until the cabbage is wilted.
- Then, stir in the miso paste and a good splash of soy sauce to taste.
- Add the tofu and let it stand for a few minutes.

- Serve and enjoy.

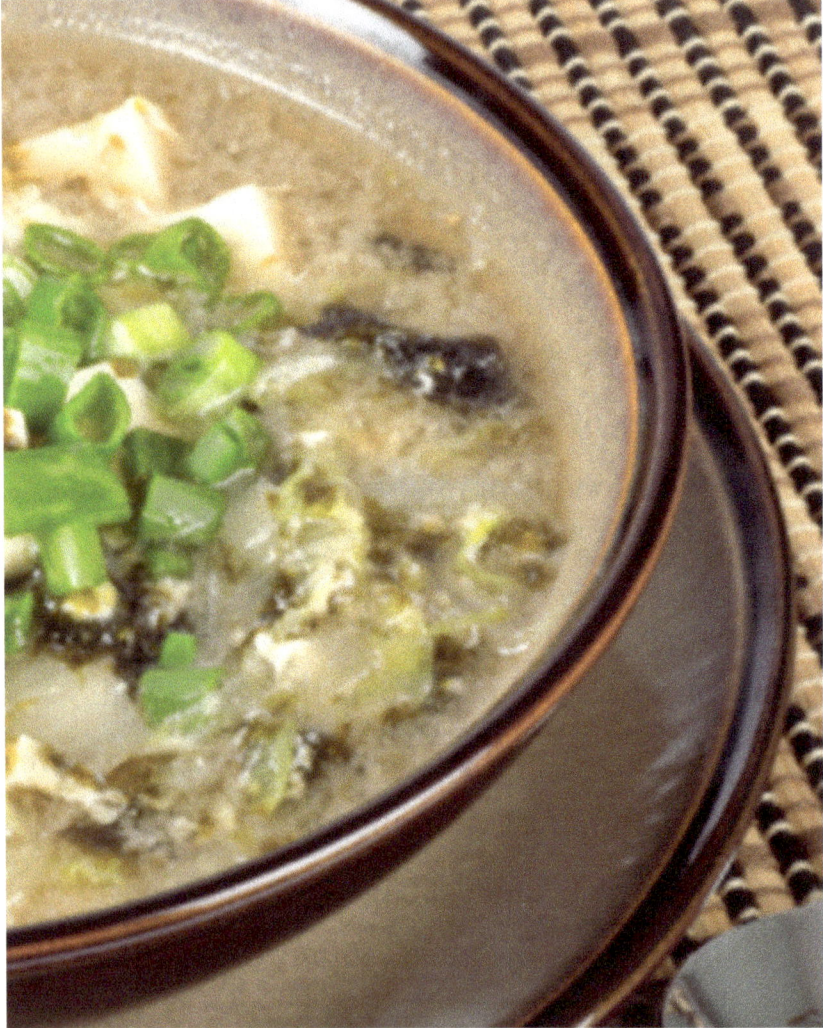

Asian inspired chicken rice balls and broth

Ingredients

- low-salt soy sauce
- 250g of mange tout
- 130g of brown rice
- 1 big bunch of coriander
- 6 spring onions
- 1 handful of beansprouts
- 4 skinless, boneless free-range chicken thighs
- 1 lime
- 2 packets of choi
- 1 stick of lemongrass
- 5cm piece of ginger
- 2 cloves of garlic
- 1 fresh red chili
- 4 kaffir lime leaves
- Sunflower oil
- 8 large raw king prawns
- 2½ tablespoons of miso paste

Directions

- Start by cooking the rice according to the packet Directions.
- Drain any excess water, let cool.
- Place leaves in a food processor with the cooled rice except coriander leaves.
- Add the onion, chicken, lemongrass, ginger, and garlic into the food processor with the kaffir lime leaves, blend until smooth.
- Transfer the mixture onto a board.
- Divide it into 16 pieces and roll each into a ball.
- Place on a plate, chill, covered, until needed.
- Place a large casserole pan over a medium-high heat.
- Add a splash of sunflower oil. Fry the rice balls for 5 minutes, or until golden brown.
- Add prawns to the pan, stir-fry for 1 minute.
- Then, stir in the miso paste with boiling water, let simmer for 10 minutes.
- Add Pak choi cut to 6 pieces with halved mange tout to the pan for the last 2 minutes.
- Stir in the beansprouts for the last 30 seconds.

- Season with a splash of soy sauce.
- Serve and enjoy.

Watercress soup

Ingredients

- 400ml of organic stock
- 2 potatoes
- 3 bunches of watercress
- 2 onions
- Olive oil
- 2 cloves of garlic

Directions

- In a large saucepan, heat bit of olive oil.
- Sauté the potato with onion and garlic until the onions are translucent.
- Add the stock and simmer until the potato is soft.
- Add chopped watercress, let simmer for 4 minutes.
- Liquidize the soup until smooth in a blender.
- Serve and enjoy with a swirl of crème fraiche.

Simple noodle soup

Ingredients

- 300g of ready-prepared rice vermicelli
- 4 spring onions
- 1 splash of soy sauce
- 1 stick of lemongrass
- 2 cloves of garlic
- 225g of raw frozen prawns
- ½ a lime
- 2 fresh red chilies
- A few sprigs of fresh coriander
- 1 liter of organic chicken stock
- 1 bok choy

Directions

- Bring the stock to boil in a large saucepan, lower heat, let simmer.
- Add bok choy, prawns, spring onions, lemon grass, and garlic to the stock.
- Cook for briefly, until the prawns have turned pink and the bok choy has wilted.

- Divide the vermicelli between 4 bowls and ladle over the soup.
- Then, scatter the chili with the coriander on top.
- Season with soy and lime juice.
- Serve and enjoy.

Fish soup

Ingredients

- 400g of prawns
- Olive oil
- 1 small bulb of fennel
- 1 leek
- Extra virgin olive oil
- 1 bunch of fresh thyme
- 3 sticks of celery
- 1 small glass of white wine
- 1 fresh red chili
- 4 cloves of garlic
- 4 tomatoes
- 440g of white fish

Directions

- Begin by gently cooking over medium heat the fennel together with the leek, celery, most of the chili and the garlic in olive oil, until soft.
- Add 1-liter water with the wine.
- let boil, then reduce heat, simmer until vegetables are cooked.

- Add the tomatoes together with the thyme and fish.
- Once the fish turns opaque, add the prawns, let simmer for 2 minutes until prawns are cooked.
- Season to taste.
- Serve and enjoy with a drizzle of extra virgin olive oil and a scattering of fresh chili.

Parsnip, sage, and white bean soup

Ingredients

- 1 parsnip
- 1 onion
- 1 organic liter of chicken stock
- 2 large parsnips
- 2 sprigs of fresh sage
- Olive oil
- 1 x 420g tin of cannellini beans
- 1 sprig of fresh sage
- 1 fresh bay leaf

Directions

- Heat 50ml of olive oil over a medium heat.
- Cook the onion together with parsnips for 10 minutes, or until softened.
- Add the bay leaf together with the beans, sage, and stock.
- Season and let simmer for 15 minutes.
- For the crispy parsnips, preheat the oven to 400°F.

- Brush the parsnip slices and sage leaves with oil.
- Then, bake for 10 minutes, or until crispy.
- Remove and discard the bay leaf from the soup.
- Beat with a stick blender until smooth.
- Taste and adjust the seasoning accordingly.
- Serve and enjoy with a drizzle of olive oil and the parsnip crisps on top.

Pumpkin and ginger soup

Ingredients

- 125ml of coconut milk
- 1kg of pumpkin
- 1-liter organic vegetable stock
- 2 shallots
- ½ tablespoon of chili powder
- 75g of ginger
- A few sprigs of fresh herbs
- Extra virgin olive oil
- 1 lime

Directions

- Put the pumpkin together with the shallots, ginger, and bit of oil in a large saucepan, sauté until soft.
- Add the stock with coconut milk and chili powder.
- Season, bring to the boil, then let simmer for 40 minutes.
- Transfer to a food processor and blend.

- Serve and enjoy with the fresh herbs, lime juice and a splash of coconut milk.

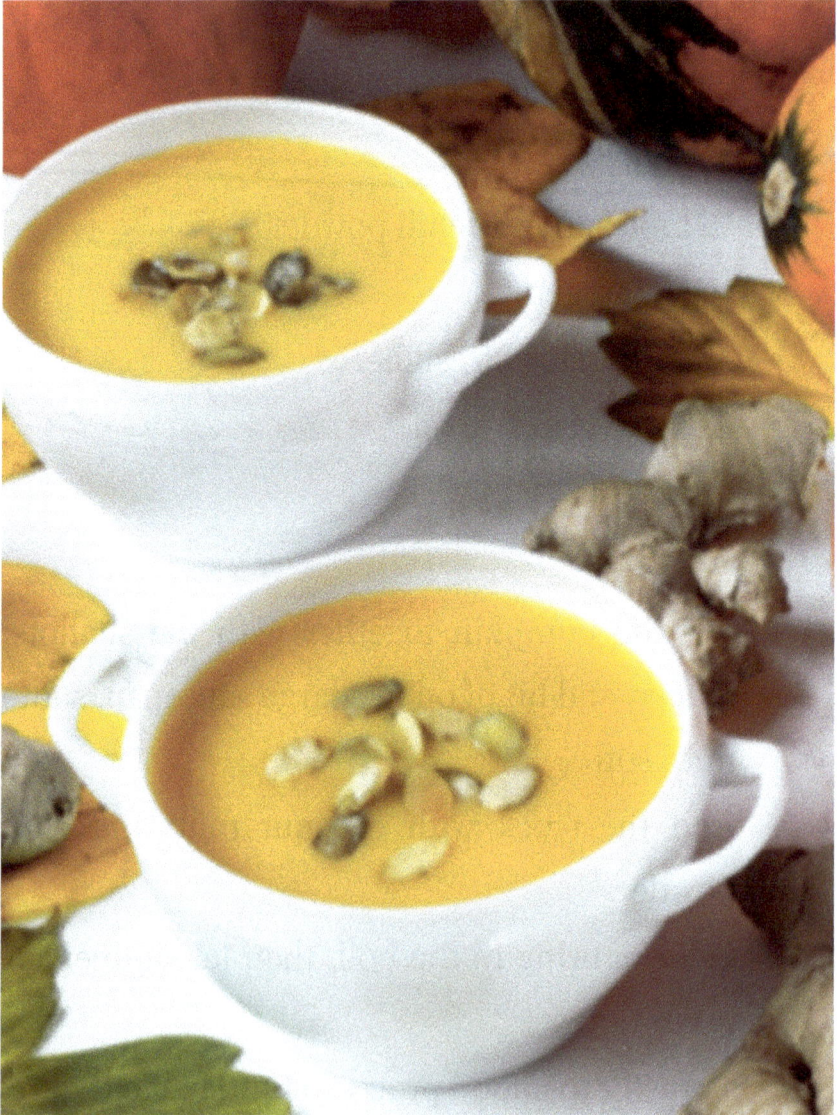

Fresh tomato broth

Ingredients

- 1 x 2kg of whole free-range chicken
- 4 onions
- 20 large ripe mixed-color tomatoes
- 1 tablespoon of tomato purée
- 6 cloves of garlic
- 4 sticks of celery

Directions

- Place the chicken together with the onions, garlic, celery, and tomatoes in a larger saucepan.
- Then, add enough cold water to cover, bring to the boil over a high heat covered for 30 minutes.
- Lower the heat when it begins to boil, let simmer over medium heat with the lid askew for 1 hour, or until the chicken is cooked through.
- Only remove the chicken and put aside.
- Sieve the soup and discard what is trapped.

- Serve and enjoy with a drizzle of basil oil, herbs.

Super tasty miso broth

Ingredients

- 1 x 200g of skinless free-range chicken breast
- 1 handful of colorful curly kale
- 20g of dried porcini mushrooms
- 1 red onion
- 1 sheet of nori
- Groundnut oil
- Rice or white wine vinegar
- 150g of mixed exotic mushrooms
- 1 x 5cm piece of ginger
- 150g of mixed brown and wild rice
- 1 heaped teaspoon miso paste
- 800ml of chicken stock
- 6 radishes

Directions

- Cook as per the package Directions. Drain.
- Rehydrate the porcini in boiling water in a small bowl,
- Place sliced onion, groundnut oil in a medium pan on a medium-high heat.

- Cook briefly until dark golden, stirring occasionally.
- Lower the heat to medium
- Add the ginger with miso paste, porcini with soaking water, and stock.
- Cover and simmer for 20 minutes.
- Toss the radishes in a splash of vinegar with a small pinch of sea salt.
- Stir through sliced chicken, torn kale, nori, broken mushroom.
- Re-cover and cook for 4 minutes. Drain and divide the rice between bowls.
- Season the broth according to your preference.
- Serve and enjoy.

www.ingramcontent.com/pod-product-compliance
Lightning Source LLC
Chambersburg PA
CBHW050746030426
42336CB00012B/1686